# Easy Cancer Cookbook for Beginners

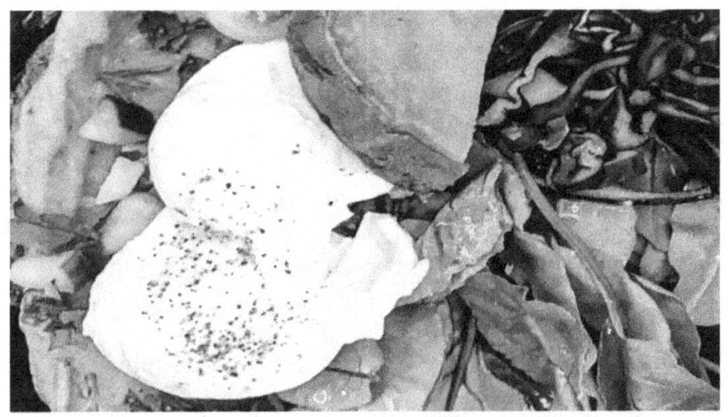

Flavorful and Nutritious Anticancer Recipes for Strength and Recovery

**Dr. Walter E. Hudson**

**Copyright by © Walter E. Hudson 2024. All rights reserved.**

# Table of content


**INTRODUCTION** ...................6

**Chapter 1** ...................8

Breakfast ........................ 8

Morning Boost Smoothie ................ 8

Nourishing Oatmeal Bowl ............10

Healthy Morning Muffins.............. 13

**Chapter 2** .................... 18

Lunch ............................ 18

Filling Lentil Soup........................ 18

Chickpea Salad Packed with Protein ..........................26

Rice Congee................................30

**Chapter 3** ....................34

Supper................................34

Delicious Stir-Fry of Vegetables 34

Gentle Baked Salmon....................38

**Chapter 4** .................... 42

Warm Soups & Broths ...........42

Chicken Noodles Soup ...................42

Nutrients Rich Vegetable Broth.51

Butternut Squash Soup with Cream..................................55

**Chapter 5**..................................**60**

Simplified Appetizers......................60

Homemade Hummus Blends.......60

Platter of Soft Cheese and Crackers...................................66

Smooth Avocado and Banana Dip.........................................70

**Chapter 6**..................................**74**

Grained Based Dish.......................74

Vegetable Pilaf with Tender Quinoa....................................74

Scrambled Egg with Brown Rice Congee...................................78

Grilled Vegetables with Soft Polenta...................................82

**Chapter 7**..................................**86**

Soft and Nutrient-Rich Main Courses..................................86

Salmon Baked in Herb Butter.....86

Softly Cooked Chicken Legs........89

Lean turkey with mashed sweet potatoes.................................93

**Chapter 8**........................................... **98**

Sweet Treats & Desserts.....................98

Chocolate Mousse with Silken Tofu ......................................................98

Energy-Boosting Banana-Oat Cookies...................................................102

Chia Seed Pudding paired with seasonal fruits.....................................106

**Chapter 9**...........................................**108**

Calm Drinks and Drinking ................. 108

Honey and Turmeric Elixir ......... 108

Calming Herbal Infusions ........... 113

Grin-Soothing Tea ....................... 116

**Conclusion**....................................... **119**

# INTRODUCTION

Every day that passes in the fight against cancer is a monument to the fortitude, resiliency, and unflinching determination of individuals who take on this terrible foe (cancer). It's a journey characterized by bravery, tenacity, and an unwavering search for hope despite obstacles.

Picture a table full of colorful, healthful food—a scene of hope and nourishment in the midst of the turbulent world of cancer therapy. Imagine the strength and flavor of each bite having the ability to transform. The narratives interwoven with the experiences of cancer patients strike a profound chord with life's fundamental qualities, highlighting the critical role nutrition plays in supporting the body and mind during these arduous times.

Thank you for visiting "Flavorful and Nutritious Anticancer Recipes for Strength and Recovery." This cookbook is a labor of love, the result of a profound understanding of the role that nutrition plays in the fight against cancer. It serves as a beacon of hope, providing approachable and simple-to-follow recipes designed for novices and recognizing the revolutionary effect of a well-nourished body on the road to healing.

This book is a source of strength and nourishment, written with one goal in mind: to give cancer patients and their loved ones a cooking partner that will not only inspire them to take up cooking again but also support them in incorporating wholesome, tasty meals into their recovery process. It's evidence for the idea that each meal has the power to lift people's spirits, impart strength, and foster optimism.

# Chapter 1

## Breakfast

### Morning Boost Smoothie

ADVICE: For happy hormones, always aim to eat between 30 or 1 hour after waking up! To reduce stress and speed up the metabolism, if you're not hungry in the morning, try a few gelatin gummies.

**Recipe**

- A handful of spinach (anti-inflammatory)
-1/2 cup of anti-inflammatory frozen blueberries.
- 1/2 cup of anti-inflammatory frozen cherries
- 1/2 cup or 3–4 frozen whole strawberries

- 1 and 1/2 cups of probiotic-rich store-bought kefir (typically strawberry flavor).

- Two tablespoons of MCT oil (a healthy fat that you might replace with avocado).

- 2 scoops of protein-rich collagen

- 1-2 scoops of electrolyte powder (I adore Organika's). I use one scoop because I think two can be a bit too strong and sweet.)

- 1/2 to 1 tsp Chlorophyll (Optional; I puree the smoothie and remove some for the kids before adding this). I add about a tsp and blend for a few more seconds to incorporate it; this works incredibly well for liver detoxification.)

Blend everything together in a blender! I would add some ice if you were using fresh fruit. Use what you have and omit the ingredient if you don't have it! Swapping simple items, like raspberries for strawberries, also works.

# Nourishing Oatmeal Bowl

**W**ith a satisfying and filling oatmeal bowl for breakfast, you can kickstart your day with a delicious meal that will nourish your body and soul. This filling dish is full of nutrition and easy on the stomach.

Total Time: 15 minutes

- Servings: 2

- Prep Time: 5 minutes

- Cook Time: 10 minutes

**Components**:

- One cup of rolled oats

- Two cups of water or non-dairy milk

- A pinch of salt

- Your preferred toppings, such as chopped fruit, almonds, seeds, honey, or cinnamon

## Kitchen Utensils

A medium-sized saucepan

- Serving bowls - Stirring spoon

## Instructions:

1. Prepare the Base:  Heat milk or water in a pot until it begins to simmer.

2. Add Oats: Mix in a little amount of salt and the rolled oats.

3. Cook:  Lower the heat and simmer the oats for five to seven minutes, stirring now and again, until they become soft and creamy.

4. Serve: Spoon the oats into dishes and top with chopped fruit, almonds, seeds, honey, or cinnamon, if preferred.

## Nutritional Information Per Serving:

- 150 calories

- 27g of carbohydrates

- 5g of protein

- 4g of fiber

- 3g of fat

## Benefits for Cancer Patients:

This filling dish of oats provides nutrients that are easily absorbed, including fiber, proteins, and carbs. It is easy on the stomach and gives long-lasting energy, making it perfect for cancer patients who have changes in appetite or digestive problems.

Concluding, this warming oatmeal bowl is a deliciously wholesome way to start your morning, providing essential nutrients and a warm hug for a brighter day ahead. Fuel your day and nurture your body with it.

## Healthy Morning Muffins

Get your day started with a tasty and nutritious boost! These satisfying and nutrient-dense Wholesome Breakfast Muffins are ideal for a leisurely morning meal.

*Total Time: 35 minutes*
*Servings: 12 muffins*
*Prep Time: 15 minutes*
*Cook Time: 20 minutes*

**Components**:

- One teaspoon of baking powder
- Two cups of whole wheat flour
- Half a teaspoon of baking soda
- 1/2 cup honey or maple syrup
- 1/4 cup heated coconut oil or olive oil
- 1/4 teaspoon salt
- Two sizable eggs
- One cup of Greek yogurt

- One tsp of vanilla extract

- A cup of carrots, grated

- 1/2 cup of chopped nuts, such as pecans, almonds, or walnuts

- 1/2 cup of dried fruit, such as chopped dates, cranberries, or raisins


**Necessary Kitchen Tools:**

- Bowls for mixing

- Muffin tin

- Cooking spray or muffin liners

- Whisk

- Oven

- Grater


## Guidelines:

1. Set the oven temperature to 175°C, or 350°F. Use cooking spray or paper liners to line a muffin tray.

2. Combine the flour, baking soda, baking powder, and salt in a sizable mixing basin.

3. Gently whisk together the eggs, Greek yogurt, honey/maple syrup, melted oil, and vanilla extract in a separate bowl.

4. Stir the dry ingredients until they are just incorporated, then gradually add the wet components.

5. Gently stir in the chopped nuts, dried fruits, and grated carrots until the mixture is well-mixed.

6. Fill each cup about two-thirds of the way to the top when spooning the batter into the muffin tin.

7. Bake for 18 to 20 minutes.

8. Place the muffins on a wire rack to cool completely after they have cooled in the pan for five minutes.

## Details for Each Serving

*- 200 calories*

*- 5g of protein*

*- 30g of carbohydrates*

*- 7g of fat*

*- 3g of fiber.*

## How Cancer Patients Can Benefit From It:

These muffins for breakfast provide a healthy, friendly alternative for those receiving cancer treatment. Enriched with whole grains, Greek yogurt's protein, and elements found in carrots, almonds, and dried fruits, they offer vital nutrients and energy that can help patients meet their dietary requirements while undergoing treatment.

***Final Thought***: These Wholesome Breakfast Muffins will give you a cozy start to the day. Not only do they add a delicious taste, but they also supply the necessary nutrients and energy for a productive morning, which makes them a great option for breakfast when things are tough.

# Chapter 2

## Lunch

### Filling Lentil Soup

Full of veggies, fresh herbs, and lentils, lentil soup is rich and filling. An excellent recipe for vegan soup that's perfect for meal planning!

*Prep: Time: 20 minutes*

*Cooking Time: 20 minutes*

*In all, 40 minutes*

With a lot of fresh herbs, veggies, and lentils, this soup is rich and filling. An excellent recipe for vegan soup that's perfect for meal planning!

## Ingredients:

- 3 tablespoons olive oil

- 1 diced onion

- 4 minced garlic cloves

- 2 tablespoons tomato paste

- 2 finely chopped carrots

- 2 finely chopped celery ribs

- 5 cups stock

- 1 cup dry, uncooked brown lentils

- Six fresh thyme sprigs (or one teaspoon dried thyme leaves)

- Two fresh rosemary sprigs

- One bay leaf

- one teaspoon salt

- One small lemon juice

## Guidelines

- Heat the oil in a medium-sized pot over medium heat.

- Add the onion and stir-fry for about 7 minutes, or until transparent.

- After adding, saute the garlic for one minute.

- Cook for 2 to 3 minutes after adding the tomato paste and stirring to coat the onions and garlic.

- Stir in the lentils, celery, carrots, bay leaf, thyme, and rosemary.

- Once the lentils are softened to your desired consistency, cook them for 35 to 40 minutes while covered, reducing heat, and simmering.

- After removing the bay leaves and herbs, purée. Add the lemon juice and stir.

Have fun!

Advice: Instant Pot

- Using the Instant Pot's sauté function, proceed as directed above.

- After 15 minutes of pressure cooking, there will be a 10-minute natural pressure release.

- Eliminate the bay leaf and herb stems, incorporate lemon juice, and then use an immersion blender to pulse three to four times.

## Storage

- For up to four days, store in the refrigerator in an airtight container.
- Can be freezed for up to six months.

## Tips for Preparing the Meal

Tomato paste: To get rid of the "canned" flavor, make sure you sauté the paste. The remaining tomato paste can be frozen in an ice cube tray and used in a different recipe.

Lentils: Dried brown lentils were used specifically for this recipe. Red lentils or cooked canned lentils are not something I suggest utilizing.

Meal prep: This dish stores incredibly well! Keep chilled for a maximum of four days and freeze for a maximum of three months.

To puree or not to purée: After cooking, pulse this soup rapidly with an immersion blender to help it thicken up. This is completely optional.

## Can I use the Instant Pot to cook this soup?

You could, I'm sure, but I haven't tried. Ten minutes at high pressure and ten minutes of natural pressure release, I would guess.

## Regarding the slow cooker, what are your thoughts?

You could, I'll wager! I would check on the lentils and try low for six to eight hours.

## What can be served with this soup?

Serving with crusty bread for dipping is something we adore. Crackers would be fantastic as well!

## Which Ingredients Are Necessary?

Lentils: For this recipe, use brown lentils rather than red ones. Unlike red lentils, they maintain their shape and don't get as soft. Learn the distinctions between red, green, and brown lentils right here!

Vegetables—carrots and celery are chopped finely—aromatics—onion and garlic contribute to flavor

Herbs: Tomato paste adds a little something to this soup. Fresh rosemary and thyme work well in this dish, and bay leaves also give some flavor.

Lemon: Squeeze in a lemon at the very end to add the acidity that enhances all the flavors. even more

Stock: Homemade bone broth or vegetarian stock, if you're not vegan.

## Information on Nutrition

- Calories: 210.89 kcal
- 27.72g of carbohydrates
- 9.15g of protein
- 7.48g of fat
- 1.05g of saturated fat
- 00.29 mg of potassium
- 11.26g of fiber
- 4.97g of sugar
- 4015.2 IU of vitamin A
- 7.77 mg of vitamin C
- 43.77 mg of calcium

- 2.92 mg of iron is included in one serving (6 batches).

# Chickpea Salad Packed with Protein

This colorful, flavor-bursting, protein-packed chickpea salad is a filling treat that is high in plant-based protein. Designed with cancer patients in mind, this light lunch option will give you the energy and vital nutrition you need to get through treatment.

*Total Time: 15 minutes*
*Servings: 4*
*Prep Time: 15 minutes*

**Components:**
- Two cans of washed and drained chickpeas (15 ounces each).
- 1 cup chopped cherry tomatoes
- 1 diced cucumber
- 1/2 finely chopped red onion

- 1/4 cup chopped fresh parsley

- 1/4 cup finely chopped fresh mint leaves

- 1/4 cup crumbled feta cheese (optional)

- One lemon's juice

- Three tsp extra virgin olive oil

- To taste, add salt and pepper.

**Utensils for the Kitchen**:

Cutting board, knife, serving bowl, whisk, and mixing bowl

**Guidelines**:

1. Combine the chickpeas, cucumber, red onion, parsley, mint, and cherry tomatoes in a mixing dish.

2. In a small bowl, mix lemon juice, olive oil, salt, and pepper.

3. Drizzle the dressing over the combination of chickpeas and gently toss until thoroughly mixed.

4. If using, sprinkle crumbled feta cheese over top.

5. Present cold in a dish.

**Information Per Serving**:

- There are 275 calories.

- 10g of protein

- 25g of carbohydrates

- 15g of fat

- 7g of fiber

**Its Benefits for Cancer Patients:**

This Chickpea Salad, Packed with Protein, provides an abundance of nutrients that are essential for cancer patients. A fantastic source of plant-based protein that supports the immune system and helps rebuild muscles is chickpeas. Furthermore, fresh veggies' vitamins and antioxidants support general wellness during this trying period.

Finally, enjoy this light lunch option of Chickpea Salad, which will give you the protein and nutrition you need to get through the day, along with a variety of flavors and textures to brighten your spirits as you recuperate.

# Rice Congee

**A** classic Asian cuisine that is both calming and comforting, rice congee is like a soft hug for the spirit. This congee is a comforting and nourishing dish that is perfect for anyone going through the difficult journey of cancer treatment because of its straightforward ingredients and delicate preparation.

*Total Time: 1 hour 10 minutes*
*Servings: 4*
*Prep Time: 10 minutes*
*Cook Time: 1 hour*

## Components:
- One cup of jasmine rice or long-grain rice.
- 8 cups chicken or vegetable broth
- Peeled and thinly sliced ginger root (one inch)
- Salt to taste

- Optional toppings: chopped scallions, cilantro, soft-boiled egg, crispy fried shallots, and shredded chicken

## Necessary Kitchen Tools:

- Big saucepan

- Knife

- Cutting board

- Wooden spoon

## Detailed Step-by-Step Guide:

1. Run cold water over the rice until the water flows clear.

2. Place the ginger pieces, broth, and washed rice in a big pot. Heat until it boils on high heat.

3. Lower the heat to a simmer and allow the congee to simmer gently for approximately an hour, or until the mixture thickens and takes on the consistency of porridge, stirring now and then to avoid sticking.

4. Take out the ginger slices and add salt to taste in the congee.

## Information Per Serving:

- 180 calories

- 40g of carbohydrates

- 4g of protein

- Fat: 1 gram

- 1g of fiber

## The Benefits of This Soup for Cancer Patients:

With its soft, readily digestible texture, rice congee offers comfort and vital nutrients. It is a calming option for cancer patients because of its mild nature, which can help with digestion and provide nutrition.

Finally, serve this hearty and soothing Rice Congee with your preferred toppings—maybe some soft-boiled eggs or shredded chicken—for a filling and soothing lunch that provides solace and nourishment during trying times.

# Chapter 3

## Supper

### Delicious Stir-Fry of Vegetables

This flavorful vegetable stir-fry is a lovely recipe that not only tantalizes the taste senses but also nourishes the body with an array of nutrients that fight cancer. Savor a burst of brilliant flavors and nutritious goodness.

*Total Time: 25 minutes*

*Servings: 4*

*Prep Time: 15 minutes*

*Cook Time: 10 minutes*

## Components:

- Two teaspoons of olive oil

- Two minced garlic cloves

- One sliced onion

- Two cups of broccoli florets

- One sliced red bell pepper

- One sliced yellow bell pepper

- One cup of clipped snow peas

- One chopped carrot

- One cup of sliced mushrooms

- Soy sauce (one tablespoon)

- One teaspoon of sesame oil

- One tablespoon of rice vinegar

- To taste, add salt and pepper.

- Optional: To garnish, add 1 tablespoon of sesame seeds to cooked brown rice or quinoa before serving.


## Necessary Kitchen Tools:

- A big skillet or wok

- A cutting board and a knife

- A wooden spatula or spoon

## Guidelines:

1. In the wok, warm up the olive oil over medium-high heat. Add the onion and minced garlic, and stir-fry until aromatic and transparent.

2. Add the bell peppers, broccoli, carrots, snow peas, and mushrooms. Vegetables should be stir-fried for 4–5 minutes to make them crisp but soft.

3. Combine the sesame oil, rice vinegar, and soy sauce in a small bowl. After adding the sauce to the veggies, mix constantly for a further one to two minutes.

4. Adjust the seasoning with salt and pepper to taste. If desired, add some sesame seeds.

5. Present the Tasty Vegetable Stir-fry on top of cooked quinoa or brown rice.

## Per Serving Nutritional Data:

- 150 calories

- 7g of total fat

- 20g of carbohydrates

- 5g of fiber

- 5g of protein

## Its Benefits for Cancer Patients:

This stir-fried vegetable dish is high in fiber, vitamins, and antioxidants that help the body fight cancer. The wide variety of vibrant veggies offers crucial nutrients that support immune system function and general health and energy.

Concluding, Enjoy this tasty vegetable stir-fry as a family around the table. It's a filling supper that not only tastes good but also nourishes the body, making it a great method to maintain health during trying times.

## Gentle Baked Salmon

Savor a mildly flavorful meal with our Gentle Baked Salmon, which is designed to comfort and nourish you when things are hard. This recipe provides warmth and critical nutrients at the same time. It's packed with omega-3s and easy on the mouth.

*Total Time: 30 minutes*
*- Servings: 4*
*-Prep Time: 10 minutes*
*- Cook Time: 20 minutes*

**Components**:
- Four of 6-oz salmon filets
- Two teaspoons of olive oil
- Two minced garlic cloves
- One sliced lemon
- Chopped fresh dill (for garnish)
- To taste, add salt and pepper.

## Utensils for the Kitchen:

- Baking dish

- Cooking brush

- Aluminum foil

- A chopping board and knife

## Guidelines:

1. Turn the oven on to 375°F, or 190°C. Use aluminum foil to line a baking dish.

2. Put the salmon filets into the baking dish that has been ready. Use salt and pepper to season each filet.

3. Combine the minced garlic and olive oil in a small bowl. Apply a layer of this blend onto the salmon filets.

4. For extra taste, place a few lemon slices on top of each filet.

5. Bake for 15 to 20 minutes, or until a fork can easily pierce the salmon, in a preheated oven.

6. Finish by adding some freshly chopped dill as a garnish.

## Per Serving Nutritional Information:

- 300 calories

34g of protein

- 17g of fat

- 2g of carbohydrates

- 1g of fiber

## Its Benefits for Cancer Patients:

This mildly baked salmon supports the body's demands during treatment by providing readily digested protein and good lipids. In addition to helping to reduce inflammation, omega-3 fatty acids may also help control nausea and other side symptoms that are frequently encountered after cancer treatments.

In conclusion, present this recipe for Gentle Baked Salmon as a nourishing and comfortable supper alternative. It offers vital nutrients and a gentle dietary experience for individuals coping with the difficulties of cancer treatment.

# Chapter 4

## Warm Soups & Broths

### Chicken Noodles Soup

*10 minutes for preparation*

*Cooking Time: 30 minutes*

*40 minutes in total*

*Six servings*

Nothing warms you up from the inside out like homemade chicken noodle soup, whether you're feeling under the weather or you just need a little comfort. In just 40 minutes, you can have the tastiest chicken noodle soup of your life on the table with this quick recipe.

## Items for Chicken Noodle Soup

The following ingredients are needed to make this delicious chicken noodle soup recipe:

Onions and Celery: Diced onions and chopped celery are sautéed in butter until fragrant and tender in the first step of this recipe for chicken noodle soup.

Broth: A combination of chicken and vegetable broths is used in this recipe for chicken noodle soup. You can just use one or the other if you're pressed for time or ingredients.

Chicken: Obviously, chicken is necessary. For a less expensive option, you can substitute cooked chicken breasts with any leftover rotisserie chicken.

Noodles: Cooking the noodles for an extended period of time will result in mushy noodles, so be careful while adding them.

Carrots: Added at the end of cooking to maintain their crispness, carrots add a burst of vibrant color and flavor. If you like your carrots tender, you can add them right at the beginning of the sautéed vegetables.

Basil and Oregano: This chicken noodle soup dish is enhanced with the warm, earthy flavor of dried basil and oregano.

## Components

- One spoonful of butter
- ½ cup finely chopped onion
- ½ cup finely chopped celery
- Four of 14.5-oz cans of chicken broth

- One 14.5-oz can of vegetable broth

- Half a pound of cooked chicken breast, chopped

- A quarter cup of noodles

- One cup of carrots, sliced

- One-half teaspoon of dried basil

- One-half teaspoon of dry oregano

- Add the ground black pepper and salt to taste.

## Guidelines

Step 1:

Melt butter in a large pot over medium heat.. Add the onion and celery and simmer for about 5 minutes or until just soft.

Step 2: Add the carrots, basil, oregano, egg noodles, chicken, vegetable broth, salt, and pepper. After combining, stir and bring to a boil.

Step 3: Simmer for 20 minutes on low heat.

## *Nutrition Information (per serving)*

162 calories

12g Carbs, 13g Protein, and 6g Fat

## How to Cook Soup with Chicken Noodles

The complete recipe is provided below, but before you start, consider these pointers for making this traditional chicken noodle soup:

### The Best Noodles for Soup (Chicken Noodle)

The classic option for chicken noodle soup is egg noodles. You could also use rotini or fusilli, but in a pinch, you could use whatever you happen to have on hand.

### Tailor to Taste

This recipe for fast chicken noodle soup is so simple that we adore it. But you may be inventive when it comes to flavors and spices. According to reviews, they enjoy adding thyme, bay leaves, garlic, and  de Provence.

## Making Do With Ingredients You Currently Own

This recipe is adaptable to easy, affordable alternatives. Try substituting oil for butter, water, and bouillon cubes for broth, or rotisserie chicken for cooked chicken breasts.

## What Pairs with Chicken Noodle Soup?

As chicken noodle soup is a meal unto itself, you really don't need to serve it with any sides—well, save perhaps some saltine crackers. To truly indulge, consider preparing a bread-based dish to absorb the rich and flavorful broth. Here are a few delectable choices:

· Toasted Garlic Bread
· Classic Dinner Rolls
· French Baguettes
· Grilled Cheese Sandwich

### How to Keep Soup with Noodles

Keep any leftover chicken noodle soup refrigerated for three to four days, sealed in an airtight container.

### Is Chicken Noodle Soup Freezable?

Indeed! If you don't intend to have the chicken noodle soup in a few days, you should freeze it. If you are planning to freeze this recipe, you might want to make the noodles and soup separately. When thawed, frozen noodles will disintegrate and get mushy.

Pour serving-size amounts of the cooled soup into freezer bags marked with the date in order to freeze chicken noodle soup, either with or without the noodles. For up to six months, freeze. Turn the stove back on.

## How Chicken Noodles Soup Aids Cancer Patients

There's no denying that a warm bowl of this aromatic soup will cheer you up, and some study even suggests that chicken noodle soup may have some medical benefits for fighting off a cold. In one study, neutrophil activity was compared against commercially available soup and homemade chicken soup. White blood cells called neutrophils aid the body in the fight against infections. In reaction to injury, infection, and inflammation, neutrophil counts and motility rise. Neutrophils moved less when the handmade and store-bought soups were present, according to the study's researchers, which may have an anti-inflammatory effect. Chicken noodle soup is full of healthful components that are great for people with colds, even if they were unable to identify the exact element in the soup that would be helpful.

The heated broth can help clear congestion in the nose and open up airways. As for "increasing nasal mucus velocity"—basically, clearing away a stuffy nose—an earlier study revealed that hot chicken soup was superior to cold water. The veggies offer anti-inflammatory vitamins like vitamin C, the chicken's protein and zinc support a stronger immune system, and the noodles taste wonderful in addition to providing energy from carbohydrates!

## Nutrients Rich Vegetable Broth

**N**utrient-rich vegetable broth is a calming elixir that is intended to support strength and vitality during difficult times. It is a blend of nourishment and healing. Packed with minerals and vitamins, this soup is a mild yet effective ally to boost immunity and facilitate digestion.

*15 minutes for preparation*
*One and a half hours of cooking*
*1 hour 45 minutes in total*
*6–8 servings*

### Ingredients:

- Quartered onions
- Chopped carrots
- Chopped celery stalks
- Chopped leek
- Sliced and trimmed
- Chopped parsnip

- One tablespoon of whole peppercorns

- One handful of fresh parsley

- Eight cups of water

- With salt to taste

**Necessary Kitchen Tools:**

A large stockpot, cheesecloth or a sieve with fine mesh, and a ladle

**Detailed Step-by-Step Guide:**

1. Fill the stockpot with the chopped veggies, parsley, and peppercorns.

2. Add the water and cook the mixture over medium-high heat until it boils.

3. To allow the flavors to mingle, reduce heat to low and boil the soup for one and a half to two hours.

4. Remove the particles from the broth by straining it through cheesecloth or a fine-mesh strainer.

5. Add salt to taste, then allow it to cool before putting it in sealed jars.

## Information Per Serving:

- Cup of serving size

- 15 Calories

- 3g of carbohydrates

- 1g of fiber

- 0.5g of protein

- Fat: 0 g

- 80% DV for vitamin A

- 10% DV for vitamin C

- Iron: 2% DV

## The Benefits of the Soup for Cancer Patients:

This highly nutritious vegetable soup provides readily assimilated nutrients, supports hydration, and provides vital vitamins and minerals that are critical for individuals receiving cancer therapy. This soup's mild flavor helps ease gastrointestinal distress, replenish fluids, and provide support during trying times.

Finally, The nutrient-rich vegetable broth is proof of the ability of basic yet effective substances to heal. It acts as a soothing elixir to help and strengthen patients facing the hardships of cancer treatment thanks to its wide array of nutrients and reassuring warmth.

## Butternut Squash Soup with Cream

This creamy butternut squash soup, with its golden tone, is silky and cozy. It is a mild treat that is ideal for nourishing the body and spirit. It is full of nutrients and has calming flavors.

*Total Time: 55 minutes*

*Servings: 4*

*Prep Time: 15 minutes*

*Cook Time: 40 minutes*

**Components**:

- One medium butternut squash (peeled and cubed)

- One chopped onion

- Two minced garlic cloves

- 4 cups chicken or veggie broth

- 1/2 teaspoon powdered nutmeg

- 1 teaspoon dried thyme

- To taste, add salt and pepper.

\- Use two teaspoons of olive oil.

\- An optional garnish Toasted pumpkin seeds, cream, or fresh parsley

**Necessary Kitchen Tools:**

\- Big pot

\- Regular blender or immersion blender

\- Wooden spoon

\- A chopping board and knife

\- Ladle

**Detailed Step-by-Step Guide:**

1. Take a big pot and heat the olive oil over medium heat. Add the chopped onion and cook for about five minutes, or until transparent.

2. Include the ground nutmeg, chopped garlic, cubed butternut squash, dry thyme, salt, and pepper. Cook for a further five minutes while stirring.

3. Add the chicken or vegetable broth and slowly bring it to a boil. Once the squash is soft, reduce heat, cover, and simmer for 20 to 25 minutes.

4. Puree the soup until it's smooth and creamy either using an immersion blender or moving it in stages to a standard blender.

5. If you are using a traditional blender, return the soup to the stove. If necessary, adjust the seasoning, then simmer for a further five minutes.

6. Spoon the rich soup into individual bowls and, if preferred, top with toasted pumpkin seeds, a swath of cream, or a sprinkling of fresh parsley.

**Information Per Serving:**

- 150 calories

- 30g of carbohydrates

- 3g of protein

- 4g of fat

- 5g of fiber

## The Benefits of the Soup for Cancer Patients:

For cancer sufferers, this Creamy Butternut Squash Soup is a nourishing and mild alternative. Rich in vitamins and antioxidants, it is easy to digest and nourish while supporting general well-being and strength maintenance during treatment.

In conclusion, This Creamy Butternut Squash Soup is comforting and nourishing in addition to being a palate-pleaser. It's a great option for people looking to add something calming and nourishing to their meals, especially during trying times, because of its rich flavors and gentle nature.

# Chapter 5

## Simplified Appetizers

## Homemade Hummus Blends

You're really missing out if you haven't begun creating your own homemade hummus. It's quick—just five minutes—and you can customize the flavor to your exact preferences. Best of all, you can manufacture a new flavor every week to keep things interesting! You won't ever go back to store-bought hummus after making your first batch at home, I swear.

**HUMMUS**: What is it?

Middle Eastern hummus is a spread or dip made from chickpeas that just requires a few basic

Ingredients. Hummus comprises, at its most fundamental level:

- Salt
- Lemon
- Garlic
- Olive Oil
- Chickpeas

*Servings 6 (each with 1/4 cup)*
*Prep in five minutes.*
*A total of five minutes*

## Ingredients

- One 15-oz can of chickpeas

- Two tsp olive oil

- 1/4 cup of lemon juice

- One-fourth cup tahini

- One garlic clove

- Salt, 1/2 tsp

- 1/4 tsp ground cumin

## DIRECTIONS

• Empty out the chickpeas. Toss in the drained chickpeas, olive oil, lemon juice, tahini, garlic, salt, and cumin in a food processor.

• Once the mixture is reasonably smooth, pulse it. Add a couple of tablespoons of water, more olive oil, or the liquid from the canned chickpeas if the mixture is too dry to process smoothly.

• After tasting the hummus, taste and add more salt, cumin, garlic, or lemon as desired.

## EQUIPMENT

Pyrex glass meal prep; food processor

**Take note**: Approximately 1.75 to 2 cups of chickpeas

## Nutrition

- 1 Serving

- Energy: 201.53 kcal

- 18.55g of carbohydrates.

- Protein: 7.4g

- Fat: 11.5g

- Sodium: 371.85mg

- Fiber: 5.92g

## How to use Hummus

Hummus is fantastic to keep in the fridge to eat as a snack with some pita bread, naan, vegetables, or chips, but it also makes a great spread for sandwiches, wraps, and loaded flatbreads. I think it's a terrific alternative to mayo or cheese because it has a really nice richness and adds moisture. I also like to use hummus as an ingredient on pizza, in place of pasta sauce, or even on scrambled eggs!

## The Span of Homemade Hummus?

Store homemade hummus in the refrigerator for up to five days. Since homemade hummus doesn't contain preservatives like certain store-bought varieties do, you should only make as much as you can consume in five days.

## Can I Use Something Other Than Tahini?

I strongly advise avoiding making hummus with tahini instead. Although a lot of people replace the tahini with either peanut butter or almond butter, the flavors of this butter are extremely different from the tahini, so this will undoubtedly alter the final flavor of your hummus. Tahini is a must if you want that real, authentic hummus taste.

## Can I Use A Blender To Make Hummus

Although some of the most potent blenders on the market, such as the Vitamix or Blentec, can prepare homemade hummus, many blenders may not be able to handle its thickness. I advise making your hummus in a food processor. However, a powerful, pricey food processor is not necessary.

## Platter of Soft Cheese and Crackers

A tasty appetizer known for its rich flavors and soft texture is the Soft Cheese and Crackers Platter. This straightforward yet sophisticated dish provides both warmth and sustenance, making it ideal for individuals looking for a light and readily digested meal starter.

*Total Time: 15 minutes*

*Servings: 4*

*Prep Time: 15 minutes*

**Components**:

- A variety of soft cheeses, including goat, camembert, and brie
- Choice of crackers (low-sodium, gluten-free, or whole grain varieties)
- Fresh fruit, such as figs, berries, or grapes
- Nuts like walnuts, cashews, and almonds

- Fruit preserves or honey (optional)

## Necessary Kitchen Tools:

- A cheese spreader or knife

- A serving board or platter

- Tiny bowls for preserves and nuts, if desired

- A chopping board and knife for preparing fruit

## Guidelines:

1. Evenly distribute the several soft cheeses, making sure they have distinct flavors and textures, onto the presentation dish or board.

2. Arrange the crackers so that they are easily accessible next to the cheeses.

3. To provide some variation to the cheese and crackers, scatter tiny bowls of nuts and preserves among them if used.

4. To enhance the cheese flavors, add fresh fruits like figs or grapes.

5. You can optionally add a little sweetness to some cheeses by drizzling them with honey.

## Information Per Serving:

This appetizer provides a combination of carbohydrates, healthy fats, and protein. Nuts contribute extra protein and healthy fats, while soft cheeses are a wonderful source of calcium and protein. This platter is nutrient-rich and delightful due to the fresh fruits' contribution of vitamins and antioxidants.

## Benefits for Cancer Patients:

The Soft Cheese and Crackers Platter is a great appetizer for anyone receiving cancer treatment because it is mild in taste. It helps to maintain nutritional balance during this difficult period by providing a source of energy and vital nutrients through its smooth textures and nutrient-dense components.

In conclusion, This appetizer offers comfort and nourishment in every mouthful, making it more than simply a fun way to start a meal. It's a smart and filling option for anyone looking for a mild yet flavorful start to their dining experience.

## Smooth Avocado and Banana Dip

With the health of cancer patients in mind, this creamy, nutrient-dense snack is called Avocado and Banana Smooth Dip. Brimming with readily assimilable components and vital vitamins, it provides a mildly aromatic complement to their nutritional and restorative journey.

*Total Time: 10 minutes*
*Servings: 4*
*Prep Time: 10 minutes*

### Components:

- One mature avocado

- One mature banana

- Two tsp Greek yogurt

- One tablespoon of juiced lemon

- Season with salt and pepper to taste

- Add a dash of paprika or cayenne pepper for a little zing

## Utensils for the Kitchen:

- Food processor or blender
- Mixing bowl - Serving spoon

## Detailed Step-by-Step Guide:

1. Preparation: Chop the banana and avocado into chunks after peeling and pitting them.

2. Blending: Put the avocado, banana, Greek yogurt, lemon juice, salt, and pepper in a food processor or blender.

3. Blend Until Smooth: Process the ingredients in a blender until a creamy consistency is achieved.

4. Season to Taste: Taste and adjust with more salt, pepper, or other spices if needed.

5. Chill and Serve: To allow the flavors to mingle, move the dip to a serving bowl and place it in the refrigerator for a short period of time. Present cold.

Information per Serving:

-Weight: 90

- Carbohydrates: 9

- Protein: 2

 - Fiber: 4

- Calories: 6 g

## How It Benefits Patients with Cancer

This silky, mild dip delivers a serving of good fats and easily digested nutrients, making it ideal for cancer patients. While the banana adds fiber and potassium, the avocado provides healthy fats that support digestion and provide you energy during this trying time.

## Final Thoughts

This Avocado and Banana Smoothie Dip is a delicious way to start any meal because of its creamy texture and nutrient-rich flavor. This is a nourishing and soothing option for anybody looking for light yet tasty appetizers while navigating cancer treatment, whether it is used as a dip for veggies or as a spread for crackers.

# Chapter 6

## Grained Based Dish

### Vegetable Pilaf with Tender Quinoa

Savor the mellow fusion of colorful veggies and nutty quinoa in this hearty Quinoa Pilaf. This recipe, which is full of nutrients and made to be easy on the tongue, is a satisfying and tasty dinner that is ideal for anyone looking to eat well while undergoing cancer treatment.

*Total Time: 40 minutes*

*Servings: 4*

*Prep Time:*

*15 minutes*

*Cook Time: 25 minutes*

## Components:

- 1 cup rinsed quinoa

- 2 cups reduced-sodium vegetable broth

- 1 tablespoon olive oil

- 1 chopped onion

- 2 minced garlic cloves

- 1 chopped carrot

- One sliced red bell pepper

– 1 cup florets of broccoli

- Season with salt and pepper

- Garnish with fresh herbs (optional)


## Utensils for the Kitchen:

- A wooden spoon or spatula

- A skillet or frying pan

- A medium pot with a lid

- A chopping board and knife

## Detailed Step-by-Step Guide:

1. Give the quinoa a good rinse in cold water and then drain.

2. Bring the vegetable broth to a boil in a medium saucepan.

3. Pour the boiling broth over the washed quinoa. Once the quinoa is cooked and the liquid has been absorbed, reduce heat to low, cover, and simmer for 15 to 20 minutes. Put aside.

4. In a skillet set over medium heat, warm the olive oil. Add the minced garlic and onion, and cook until transparent and aromatic.

5. Include the broccoli, red bell pepper, and sliced carrot in the skillet. Cook the vegetables for five to seven minutes, or until they are crisp and tender.

6. In the saucepan, mix the cooked vegetables and prepared quinoa. Gently stir to incorporate.

7. Add more salt and pepper to taste when seasoning. If desired, garnish with fresh herbs.

## Information Per Serving:

This Quinoa Pilaf dish is a great way to get plenty of fiber, vitamins, and minerals that are important for bolstering the immune system when undergoing cancer treatment. As a complete protein, quinoa helps to sustain muscle strength and energy levels. The blend of soft veggies provides minerals and antioxidants essential for general health.

Finally, Quinoa Pilaf and other grain-based recipes provide a nourishing and cozy choice for those going through cancer treatment. Full of critical nutrients and simple to digest, it's a tasty but moderate meal that supports general well-being during a trying period and offers necessary food.

# Scrambled Egg with Brown Rice Congee

This dish, Brown Rice Congee with Scrambled Egg, is a soothing grain dish that is especially good for cancer patients who are looking for a light and nutritious lunch. This dish provides comfort and vital nutrients during trying times because of its soft texture and nutrient-rich ingredients.

*Total Time: 1 hour*
*Servings: 4*
*Prep Time: 10 minutes*
*Cook Time: 50 minutes*

**Ingredients:**

- 1 cup brown rice

- 6 cups vegetable or chicken broth with reduced sodium

- 2 cups water

- Two beaten eggs

- One tablespoon of olive oil

- Season with salt and pepper to taste

- Add extra protein by topping with shredded chicken, sesame oil, and chopped green onions.

**Cookware**:

- A medium-sized pot

- A fork or whisk

- Ladle

- Wooden spoon or spatula

- Serving bowls

Steps: 1. Congee Preparation: Give the brown rice a good rinse. Bring the water, broth, and rice to a boil in a pot. Turn down the heat to low and simmer, partially covered, until the rice is cooked, about 40 to 45 minutes, stirring now and then.

2. Scramble Eggs: In a pan over medium heat, warm up the olive oil while the congee cooks. Add the whisked eggs and mix gradually until they become scrambled. Take off the heat.

3. Combine: After the congee is cooked, carefully add the scrambled eggs to the saucepan and stir constantly for two to three minutes, or until everything is well blended. To taste, add salt and pepper for seasoning.

4. Servings: Ladle the mildly hot congee into bowls for serving (step four). If preferred, add other toppings like shredded chicken for extra protein, chopped green onions, or a splash of sesame oil.

## Nutritional Data per Serving

: 240 calories

- 8g of protein

- 40g of carbohydrates

- 5g of fat

- 3g of fiber

## How Cancer Patients Can Benefit From This Dish

This mild but nutrient-dense congee helps sustain energy levels during treatment by providing readily digested protein and carbs. Its soft texture and nutritious ingredients make it appropriate for anyone with digestive problems or trouble swallowing.

In conclusion, Brown Rice Congee with Scrambled Egg is the epitome of warming grain dishes, providing a balance of convenience and nutrition to assist those receiving cancer treatment.

# Grilled Vegetables with Soft Polenta

This dish for Soft Polenta with Grilled Vegetables is a delicious combination of a bright array of grilled vegetables and creamy, cozy polenta that offers both flavor and health.

*45 minutes in total*

*15 minutes for preparation*

*30 minutes for cooking;*

*Serves: 4*

## Components:

- Two tablespoons butter
- Four cups chicken or veggie broth
- One cup polenta (cornmeal)
- Assorted veggies (bell peppers, zucchini, eggplant, cherry tomatoes, etc.) for grilling
- Salt and pepper to taste
- Olive oil for grilling

- Optional fresh herb garnish

**Necessary Kitchen Tools:**

- Grill or grill pan - Saucepan

- Wooden spoon

- A serving dish

**Guidelines**:

1. Bring the broth to a boil in a saucepan. Pour the polenta in gradually while whisking constantly to prevent lumps.

2. Lower the heat to low and simmer the polenta for 20 to 25 minutes, stirring now and again, or until it thickens and gets soft and creamy.

3. Add butter, season with pepper and salt, and turn off the heat.

4. In the interim, warm up the grill or grill pan. Vegetables should be grilled till soft and slightly browned after lightly brushing with olive oil.

5. Transfer the grilled veggies onto a platter or plates and top with the creamy polenta. If desired, garnish with fresh herbs.

## Information Per Serving:

- 250 calories

- 6g of total fat

- 42g of carbohydrates

- 6g of fiber

- 5g of protein

## How Cancer Patients Can Benefit From This Dish

It's a comfort food that's easy to digest and full of nutrients and is served with grilled vegetables and this soft polenta. While the colorful grilled vegetables provide a range of vitamins and antioxidants, the soft texture of polenta is soothing to delicate digestive systems and helps preserve vital nutrients throughout cancer treatment.

In conclusion - Grains-Based Dishes

For patients undergoing cancer treatment, grain-based meals like this Soft Polenta with Grilled Vegetables provide a nourishing and cozy choice. These meals, with their mild textures and adaptability, are meant to be nourishing and consoling during hard times.

# Chapter 7

## Soft and Nutrient-Rich Main Courses

### Salmon Baked in Herb Butter

Easy prep time of 15 minutes and only one pan is needed for this garlicky, buttery baked salmon. Serve fish slathered in a delicious herb butter that highlights McCormick Perfect Pinch, an Italian Seasoning. Bake till tender.

*5 minutes for preparation*

*10 minutes for cooking*

*308 calories*

*5 Ingredients*

## *Measurement*

- 1/4 cup softened butter (1/2 stick)

- McCormick Garlic Powder, 1/2 teaspoon

- Half a teaspoon of Italian seasoning from McCormick Perfect Pinch

- McCormick Ground Mustard, half a teaspoon

- One-pound filets of salmon

## Directions

1. Set oven temperature to 350°F. In a medium bowl, thoroughly mix butter, ground mustard, Italian seasoning, and garlic powder.

2.

Place the fish on a foil-lined shallow baking tray. Apply the herb butter mixture to the fish.

3.

When the fish flakes easily with a fork, bake it for 10 minutes for every inch of thickness.

## INFO ON NUTRITION (per Serving)

- 308 calories

- 24g total fat, 102 mg cholesterol

- 150 milligrams of sodium

- 0g of carbs, 0g of fiber

- 23g of protein.

## Softly Cooked Chicken Legs

**T**aste the succulent perfection of Braised Chicken Thighs - a nutritious and flavorful dish perfect for those hard times.

*Total Time: 1 hour 45 minutes*
*Servings: 4*
*Prep Time: 15 minutes*
*Cook Time: 1 hour 30 minutes*

**Components**:

- Four skin-on, bone-in chicken thighs

- Two teaspoons of olive oil

- One chopped onion

- Three minced garlic cloves

- One cup chopped tomatoes

- One cup chicken broth

- A teaspoon of thyme, dried

- Season with salt and pepper

- Garnish with finely chopped fresh parsley.

## Utensils for the Kitchen

- Tongs - Wooden spoon

- Deep skillet or Dutch oven with lid

- Chef's knife

- A chopping block

## Guidelines:

1. Season chicken thighs extensively with salt and pepper.

2. Season chicken thighs extensively with salt and pepper. Place the skin-side-down chicken thighs on top and fry until golden brown. Turnover and grill the other side. Take out and place aside.

3. Saute onions in the same saucepan until they become transparent. Once added, cook for a further minute.

4. Add diced tomatoes and chicken broth. Simmer after adding the dried thyme.

5. Put the chicken thighs back in the saucepan, cover it, and simmer it on low heat for an hour, or until it is cooked through and soft.

6. Garnish with chopped parsley and serve hot.

## Each Serving:

- Calories 320 kcal

- 25 g of protein

- 5 g of carbohydrates

- 22 g of fat

- 5 g of saturated fat

- 140 mg of cholesterol

- 350 mg of sodium

- 1 g of fiber

- 2 g of sugar.

## How Does It Help?

This is a high-protein dish that can help you stay strong while undergoing cancer treatment. It is easy to chew and digest because of the tenderness that is ensured by the gentle braising method. It offers patients a nourishing and pleasant option because of the additional nutrients from tomatoes and aromatics.

In addition to being a tasty dish, braised chicken thighs are a nutrient-dense main course that is intended to assist those receiving cancer treatment by giving them the comfort and critical food they need as they heal.

## Lean turkey with mashed sweet potatoes

This filling and healthy recipe blends lean, high-protein turkey with the earthy sweetness of mashed sweet potatoes to create a satisfying and complete dinner.

*Total Time: 45 minutes*
*Servings: 4*
*Prep Time: 15 minutes*
*Cook Time: 30 minutes*

**Detailed Step-by-Step Guide**:

1. Prepare Ingredients: Cut three large sweet potatoes into cubes after peeling them. Use salt, pepper, and your favorite herbs to season one pound of lean ground turkey.

2. Boil Sweet Potatoes: Put the sweet potato chunks in a pot, add water to cover, and boil for

15 to 20 minutes, or until the potatoes are soft. Empty.

3. Cook Turkey: Cook the seasoned turkey over medium heat in a separate skillet until it is browned and cooked through, which should take about ten minutes.

4. Mash Potatoes: In a basin, mash the cooked sweet potatoes until they are smooth. To taste, adjust seasoning with salt and pepper.

5. Combine: Ensure that the cooked turkey is thoroughly mixed into the mashed sweet potatoes.

**Components**:

- Three substantial sweet potatoes

- One pound of lean ground turkey

- Season with salt, pepper, and your favorite herbs

## Necessary Kitchen Tools:

A boiling pot, a skillet, and a fork or potato masher for frying turkey

## Information Per Serving:

- 280 calories

- 25g of protein

- 30g of carbohydrates

- 7g of fat

- 4g of fiber

## How This Recipe Aids Cancer Patients

This high-nutrient dish gives you the necessary amount of protein and carbohydrates for energy, and because mashed sweet potatoes are soft and easy on the stomach, they are a good choice for cancer patients receiving treatment.

Final Thoughts - Mashed Sweet Potatoes with Lean Turkey is a hearty and satisfying main dish that provides vital nutrients and tastes to help people on their path to recovery from cancer treatment.

# Chapter 8

## Sweet Treats & Desserts

### Chocolate Mousse with Silken Tofu

Enjoy this silken tofu chocolate mousse, a rich but health-conscious dessert that tantalizes the taste senses and provides an energy boost, guilt-free. Ideal for people who want a creamy pleasure when things are hard.

*Total Time: 10 minutes*

*Servings: 4*

*Prep Time: 10 minutes*

## Components:

- One 12-oz container of silken tofu; one-fourth cup of unsweetened cocoa powder
- 1/4 cup honey or maple syrup
- One teaspoon vanilla essence and one-fourth teaspoon salt
- Fresh berries, shaved chocolate, or chopped nuts are optional garnishes.

## Necessary Kitchen Tools:

- Food processor or blender
- Mixing bowl
- Presenting bowls or glasses

## Guidelines:

1. Transfer the drained silken tofu to the food processor or blender.
2. Fill the blender with salt, vanilla extract, cocoa powder, and maple syrup or honey.

3. Blend the mixture, scraping down the sides as necessary, until it's smooth and creamy.

4. Spoon mousse into dishes or glasses for serving.

5. Before serving, let the food cool in the refrigerator for at least half an hour.

6. If preferred, garnish with chopped nuts, shaved chocolate, or fresh berries.

**Information Per Serving:**

- 120 calories

- 7g of protein

- 4g of fat

- 15g of carbohydrates

- 3g of fiber

**How It Benefits Patients with Cancer**

This protein-rich and reasonably sugar-free Silken Tofu Chocolate Mousse has a smooth, pleasant texture. It's a dessert that's simple to eat due to its soft nature and important nutrients for cancer patients undergoing treatment.

In conclusion, Enjoy the deliciousness of this Silken Tofu Chocolate Mousse not only as a beautiful dessert but also as a nourishing and cozy treat that is intended to provide a brief moment of happiness and sustenance, especially for those who are looking for mild yet delectable treats during difficult times.

## Energy-Boosting Banana-Oat Cookies

These banana-oat cookies provide a pleasant burst of energy and nutrients during trying times. These sweets are made with healthy ingredients and are meant to cheer you up and give you encouragement when things get hard.

*Total Time: 25 minutes*
*Servings: 12 cookies*
*Prep Time: 10 minutes*
*Cook Time: 15 minutes*

**Detailed Step-by-Step Guide:**

1. Prepare and Heat: Set the oven's temperature to 350°F (175°C). A baking sheet should be lined with parchment paper.

2. Mash the Bananas: Mash two ripe bananas until smooth in a mixing dish.

3. Combine Substances: To the mashed bananas, add ½ cup rolled oats, ¼ cup raisins, ¼ cup chopped nuts (almonds or walnuts), 1 teaspoon cinnamon, and a dash of salt. Until all components are mixed, thoroughly mix.

4. Form Cookies: Using a spoon, scoop out portions of the mixture and transfer them to the baking sheet that has been preheated. Shape them into round cookie shapes.

5. Cake: After preheating the oven, place the baking sheet inside and bake the cookies for 15 minutes, or until they are golden brown.

6. Relax and Present: After baking, allow the cookies to cool for a few minutes on the baking sheet before moving them to a wire rack to finish cooling. Savor these delicious goodies!

## Components:

- One and a half cups rolled oats

- ¼ cup raisins

- two ripe bananas

- 1/4 cup finely chopped nuts (walnuts or almonds)

- tsp cinnamon

- A dash of salt


## Necessary Kitchen Tools:

- Parchment paper

- Baking sheet

- Mixing bowl

- Spoon

- A cooling wire rack


## Information Per Serving:

- 90 calories

- 16g of carbohydrates

- 2g of protein and 3g of fat

- 2g of fiber

## How It Benefits Patients with Cancer

The purpose of these Banana-Oat Cookies is to provide a healthy snack that is easy to chew and digest, while also offering necessary energy and fiber. The trifecta of oats, bananas, and nuts offers a steady energy source that helps patients receive cancer treatments.

Finally, beyond simply being a delicious treat, these Banana-Oat Cookies provide support and vitality during trying times. Savor these healthy treats as a guilt-free treat that uplifts the soul and the body.

# Chia Seed Pudding paired with seasonal fruits

*20 minutes for preparation*

*20 minutes in total*

*Yield: 3 cups pudding plus fruit*

*servings: 6.*

## Ingredients:

• 1 14-ounce container of light coconut milk without added sugar

• One cup of fat-free plain Greek yogurt

• Two tablespoons of pure maple syrup

• One-half teaspoon of vanilla

• Half a cup of chia seeds

• Two cups of finely diced fresh fruit or berries (strawberries, mango, pineapple, peaches, blueberries, raspberries, and/or raspberries)

• Six teaspoons of roasted, unsweetened shredded coconut.

## Guidelines

Step 1:

Mix the yogurt, maple syrup, coconut milk, and vanilla in a medium-sized bowl. Add the chia seeds and stir. Distribute the mixture among six bowls for serving. Wrap in foil and refrigerate overnight.

Step 2: Spoon fruit equally over pudding in bowls to serve. Add a little coconut.

***Nutrition Information (per serving)***

161 calories

18g Carbs

7g Protein, and 8g Fat

# Chapter 9

## Calm Drinks and Drinking

### Honey and Turmeric Elixir

This calming elixir of turmeric and honey combines the potent anti-inflammatory effects of turmeric with the inherent sweetness of honey. This reassuring beverage is intended to offer consolation as well as possible health advantages to individuals experiencing difficult times.

*5 minutes for preparation*

*10 minutes for cooking*

*15 minutes for the entire process*

*2 servings*

Components:

- One teaspoon of turmeric powder

- Two cups of water

- 1/2 teaspoon grated ginger

- 1 tablespoon honey

- A dash of black pepper

- Lemon slices (optional garnish)

## Necessary Kitchen Tools:

- Strainer

- Whisk

- Small saucepan

- Serving mugs or cups

## Detailed Step-by-Step Guide:

1. Simmer the water in a small pot until it begins to gently simmer.

2. To the simmering water, add the grated ginger, turmeric powder, and a dash of black pepper.

3. Combine the ingredients with a whisk and simmer over low heat for approximately 7-8 minutes.

4. Take the pot off of the burner and give the mixture a minute to cool.

5. After adding the honey, mix until it dissolves.

6. To serve, strain the elixir into cups or mugs.

7. You can optionally add more flavor by garnishing with a piece of lemon.

**Information Per Serving**:

- 30 kcal of calories

- 8g of carbohydrates

- Fat: 0 g

- Protein: 0 grams

- 0.5g of fiber

- Sugar (seven grams)

## Its Benefits for Cancer Patients

Because of the anti-inflammatory qualities of turmeric and the calming effects of honey, this elixir of turmeric and honey may help cancer patients. Because of its reputation for reducing inflammation, turmeric may be especially helpful for patients who are uncomfortable while undergoing therapy. Furthermore, the inherent sweetness of honey might offer solace and some alleviation.

In conclusion, this Turmeric and Honey Elixir is a calming addition to your routine that provides warmth, comfort, and the possible health advantages of its ingredients. Take a sip and accept this mild elixir as a soothing assistance on your path.

Note: Before introducing any new components to your diet, especially while receiving cancer treatment, please speak with a healthcare provider.

## Calming Herbal Infusions

**D**uring the difficult path of cancer treatment, moments of peace can be experienced by seeking comfort in a relaxing herbal infusion. During trying times, this comforting drink provides a mild break and consolation.

**Components**:

- Two teaspoons of dried chamomile flowers

- Two glasses of water

- One teaspoon of lavender buds, dried

- Honey (for sweetness; optional)

**Utensils for the Kitchen**:

- Strainer

- Teapot or heat-resistant pitcher

- Cups or mugs

## Guidelines:

1. In a pot, bring two cups of water to a boil.

2. Incorporate dried lavender buds and chamomile flowers into the boiling water.

3. Take the saucepan off of the burner and let the herbs for five to seven minutes.

4. Pour the infusion through a strainer into a heatproof pitcher or teapot.

5. Fill mugs or cups with the mixture after adding honey, if preferred.

## Details per Serving:

- Calories: Negligible

Health Benefits: The relaxing effects of chamomile and lavender are well-known; they can promote relaxation and possibly lessen tension and anxiety.

## Its Benefits for Cancer Patients:

For cancer patients, this mild herbal infusion provides a soothing break, and it may help promote calm during stressful times. During treatment, chamomile and lavender may also assist general well-being by reducing anxiety and enhancing sleep quality.

Finally, savor the solace of a soothing herbal tea, a mild concoction that provides moments of calm and repose amid trying circumstances. Take a sip and let this cozy hug of peaceful nature comfort you.

# Grin-Soothing Tea

Accept the soothing warmth of Soothing Ginger Tea, a nourishing infusion designed to offer relief and support during trying times. This tea, which is bursting with the health benefits of ginger, promises to soothe you with every sip.

## Components:

- One 1-inch piece of fresh ginger, peeled and sliced
- Two cups of water
- One tablespoon honey, if desired
- Optional garnish of lemon slices

## Utensils for the Kitchen:

- Strainer - Saucepan
- Cups or a teapot

## Guidelines:

1. Place two cups of water in a pot and gently bring to a boil.

2. To infuse the flavors, add the sliced ginger to the boiling water, lower the heat, and simmer for ten to fifteen minutes.

3. Pour the water with the ginger infusion into glasses or a teapot.

4. Garnish with a lemon slice for added zest and honey, if preferred.

## Information Per Serving:

- 10 kcal of calories

- 3 grams of carbs and 0 grams of fat

- Protein: 0 grams

- 2g of sugar

- Sodium: 1 mg

## How It Benefits Patients with Cancer

Ginger has calming and anti-inflammatory qualities that can help reduce nausea, which is a frequent side effect of cancer treatment. This mild tea is a calming cure, settling upset stomachs and offering warmth and moisture when things get tough.

Soothing Ginger Tea is a nurturing ally that provides relief and comfort with its mild warmth and healing qualities. Include this tranquil potion in your daily routine to benefit from its calming properties and maintain your well-being when things get tough.

# Conclusion

Cooking takes on a purpose beyond providing food in the complex web of fighting cancer; it becomes a source of unfathomable power, a comforting light, and a canvas for healing. Every recipe created using this cookbook is an ode to perseverance and the unwavering spirit that rises above misfortune.

At the end of "Flavorful and Nutritious Anticancer Recipes for Strength and Recovery," remember that the book was written with compassion and support for others in mind. It's more than simply a cookbook; it's a journey of healing and optimism that uses the culinary arts to reveal the way to well-being.

This recipe book is a silent pledge of assistance, a steady ally over the rough terrain of cancer treatment. It is evidence of the significant effect that healthy, thoughtful cooking can have on the body and psyche, providing not only nourishment but also a spiritual salve.

I want to thank all of the readers who have joined us on this culinary journey. The love and intention that permeate the pages of this book stem from your bravery and faith in these recipes.

Keep using the spatula with inquiry and enthusiasm. Allow your kitchen's scents to create a hopeful symphony. Investigate, try new things, and put love into every meal. This is just the beginning of your trip; there is much more exploration and growth ahead.

I hope every meal you make is an ode to health, life, and the steadfast spirit that characterizes your path. Continue to cook and to thrive.